METABOLIC APPROACH TO CANCER FOR WOMEN

Integrating Deep Nutrition and Nourishing Whole-Food to Starve Cancer with Delicious Recipes, Meal Plan and Exercise for Treatment & Recovery

Dr. Martins Sant

ABOUT THE AUTHOR

Dr. Martins Sant is not just a name; he's your dedicated partner on the journey to a healthier and happier you. With over a decade of experience as a distinguished Nutritionist and Dietitian, Dr. Sant has helped countless individuals transform their lives through the power of proper nutrition.

Armed with a Master's Degree in Nutrition, Dr. Sant's expertise extends far beyond the classroom. He combines his extensive academic knowledge with a profound passion for wellness to create practical and personalized nutrition plans that bring tangible results.

He is on a mission to empower you with the knowledge and tools to make informed dietary choices that enhance your vitality, longevity, and overall well-being. Dr. Sant understands that every person is unique, and he tailors his guidance to suit your individual needs and goals.

Whether you're looking to shed those extra pounds, manage chronic health conditions, or simply adopt a balanced and nutritious lifestyle, Dr. Martins Sant is your go-to expert. His compassionate and approachable demeanor, coupled with a deep commitment to your success, make him a trusted advisor you can rely on.

Join Dr. Sant on a journey to unlock the secrets of nourishing your body and achieving the best version of yourself. With his guidance, you'll discover that optimal health is within your reach, and a fulfilling, nutritious life is just a choice away.

TABLE OF CONTENTS

INTRODUCTION **8**

The Metabolic Theory of Cancer: An Overview.........8

Understanding Women's Unique Health Challenges .9

The Role of Diet and Exercise in Cancer Prevention 10

Chapter 1 ....**14**

Metabolism and Cancer: The Connection **14**

Defining Metabolism in the Context of Health and Disease 14

How Cancer Cells Metabolize: The Warburg Effect .16

Chapter 2 ....**19**

Nutritional Science for Women **19**

Macronutrients and Micronutrients: What Women Need 19

The Impact of Hormones on Women's Metabolism..22

Chapter 3 ....**27**

Exercise Physiology for Cancer Prevention **27**

How Physical Activity Influences Cellular Health......27

Tailoring Exercise to Women's Physiological Needs31

Chapter 4 .... **35**

Anti-Cancer Foods for Women **35**

Phytochemicals and Antioxidants: A Woman's Armor
....36

Superfoods in the Fight Against Cancer 37

Chapter 5 .... **42**

Dietary Patterns for Metabolic Health **42**

The Mediterranean Diet and Cancer Prevention 42

Relationship Between Weight Loss and Cancer in
Women 46

Pros of the Ketogenic Diet for Women's Health 48

Cons of the Ketogenic Diet for Women's Health 49

Chapter 6 .... **51**

Supplements and Women's Health **51**

Vitamins and Mineral Supplements for Women's
Health Against Cancer 51

Risks and Considerations of Vitamin and Mineral
Supplements 53

Herbs for Women Health Against Cancer 54

CHapter 7 .... **58**

Building a Cancer-Resistant Body 58

Strength Training: The Unsung Heroine 58

Cardiovascular Health: More Than Heart Deep 61

Yoga and Mind-Body Wellness 62

The Role of Stress Reduction in Cancer Prevention 63

Yoga: Harmonizing Body and Mind 65

Creating Your Personalized Exercise Plan 67

Assessing Your Fitness Level 67

Setting Realistic and Sustainable Goals 69

Weeks 1-4: Foundation Building 70

Weeks 9-12: Consistency and Growth 71

Weeks 13-16: Goal Assessment and Adjustment 71

Chapter 8 ....**72**

Implementing a Metabolic Approach Via Recipes and Meal Planning **72**

Breakfast Recipes 72

Lunch Recipes 80

Dinner Recipes 89

Snacks Recipes 95

21-Days Meal Plan 103

Chapter 9 .... **113**

Lifestyle Factors and Metabolic Health **113**

Sleep, Stress, and Cancer Risk 113

The Importance of Community and Support 115

Chapter 10 .... **117**

Beyond Prevention - A Supportive Journey **117**

Integrating Metabolic Approaches with Traditional Care 117

Navigating Treatments: A Woman's Guide 120

The Role of Nutrition in Recovery 123

Exercise in Recovery 125

Stories of Hope: Women's Experiences with a Metabolic Approach 126

Conclusion **128**

INTRODUCTION

Cancer remains one of the most formidable health challenges of our time, and its impact on women's health is particularly profound. While the battle against cancer continues on multiple fronts, a growing body of research suggests that a metabolic approach to cancer prevention and treatment may offer new hope. This book is dedicated to exploring how women can harness the power of food and exercise to influence their metabolic health and, in turn, fortify their bodies against cancer.

The Metabolic Theory of Cancer: An Overview

At the heart of this approach is the metabolic theory of cancer, a concept that has gained traction alongside the traditional genetic view. The theory posits that cancer is not just a result of genetic mutations but also a metabolic disease, where the way cancer cells process energy is fundamentally flawed. Unlike healthy cells that rely on oxidative phosphorylation for energy, cancer cells depend heavily on glycolysis, even in the presence of oxygen. This phenomenon, known as the Warburg effect, suggests that by altering the body's metabolic environment, we may be able to impact cancer cell growth.

The implications of this theory are profound for women, who often face unique metabolic challenges due to hormonal fluctuations throughout their lives. By understanding how metabolism and cancer are intertwined, women can potentially influence their cancer risk through diet and lifestyle choices. This book aims to demystify the science behind the metabolic theory of cancer, providing readers with a solid foundation to understand how their daily choices can contribute to their overall health.

Understanding Women's Unique Health Challenges

Women's bodies are complex systems influenced by a symphony of hormones that play a significant role in their metabolic health. Estrogen, progesterone, and other hormones not only regulate reproductive functions but also impact metabolism, weight, and insulin sensitivity. These hormonal variations can affect a woman's cancer risk at different stages of her life, such as during menstruation, pregnancy, and menopause.

Moreover, certain cancers, like breast and ovarian cancer, are more prevalent in women and have been linked to hormonal and metabolic factors. The interplay between hormones, metabolism, and cancer risk underscores the need for a tailored approach to cancer prevention for women—one that acknowledges the intricacies of their bodies.

In this book, we delve into the unique metabolic challenges women face and how these can be addressed through targeted dietary and exercise strategies. We explore how women can optimize their hormonal health through nutrition, how certain foods can help balance hormones naturally, and how physical activity can enhance metabolic flexibility, potentially reducing cancer risk.

The Role of Diet and Exercise In Cancer Prevention

Physical Activity and Cancer Risk Reduction

Regular physical activity is strongly associated with a decreased risk of several types of cancer. For women, the evidence is particularly compelling in the context of breast and endometrial cancers. Engaging in moderate to vigorous physical activity can act as a powerful preventive measure. The American Cancer Society recommends 150-300 minutes of moderate intensity or 75-150 minutes of vigorous intensity activity per week for adults, with an emphasis on exceeding the upper limit of 300 minutes for optimal benefits.

Impact of Exercise on Metabolic Health

Exercise influences metabolic health by improving insulin sensitivity, reducing inflammation, and helping to maintain a healthy body weight. These factors are crucial because they can affect cancer risk. For instance, obesity is a known risk factor for several types of cancer, and physical activity can help mitigate this risk by preventing weight gain.

Dietary Patterns and Cancer Prevention

A diet rich in fruits, vegetables, whole grains, and lean proteins, while low in processed foods and red meats, is often recommended for cancer prevention. Specific foods and nutrients have been identified for their potential anti-cancer properties, including dietary fiber, which is linked to a reduced risk of colorectal cancer, and phytochemicals found in a variety of plant-based foods, which may protect against various forms of cancer.

Synergistic Effects of Diet and Exercise

The combination of a nutritious diet and regular physical activity can have synergistic effects on health. Not only do they each contribute to cancer prevention, but together they can also enhance overall metabolic health, support immune function, and reduce the risk of other chronic diseases such as heart disease and diabetes.

Practical Recommendations

To integrate these findings into daily life, it is recommended to:

- Engage in regular physical activity, incorporating both aerobic and strength-training exercises.
- Follow a diet that emphasizes plant-based foods, lean proteins, and whole grains.
- Limit sedentary behaviors such as prolonged sitting or screen time.
- Gradually increase the intensity and duration of physical activity if currently inactive.

- Consult with healthcare providers before starting any new diet or exercise regimen, especially for individuals with pre-existing health conditions.

CHAPTER 1

METABOLISM AND CANCER: THE CONNECTION

Defining Metabolism in the Context of Health and Disease

The word "metabolism" refers to the vast array of biochemical reactions that power our cells' ability to survive. It is the culmination of all chemical processes that take place inside the body, transforming food and liquids into energy and the components needed for cellular development and repair. When it comes to health and illness, metabolism is a two-edged sword: when it is dysregulated, it can lead to disease, but it is also an essential function for sustaining life.

Catabolism and anabolism are the two basic pathways that make up metabolism. The process of breaking down molecules to release energy is called catabolism, and it is vital for supplying the fuel that keeps our cells running. On the other hand, anabolism uses the energy produced by catabolic processes to synthesize all the chemicals that cells require.

These metabolic processes are carefully controlled and balanced to suit the requirements of the body in a healthy condition. A perfectly synchronized metabolic response is demonstrated, for example, by the secretion of insulin after eating, which aids in the cells' absorption of glucose from the blood for energy.

On the other hand, sickness can result from an imbalance in metabolic processes. For instance, diabetes impairs the body's capacity to control blood sugar levels, frequently as a result of problems with insulin synthesis or function, which sets off a chain reaction of health problems. Comparably, metabolic dysregulation—where cancer cells modify their metabolism to facilitate fast growth and multiplication, frequently at the expense of the body's regular processes—is a defining feature of cancer.

The Warburg effect, or metabolic hypothesis of cancer, suggests that even in the presence of oxygen, malignant cells choose to produce energy through glycolysis, which is less effective than the regular oxidative phosphorylation process that healthy cells employ. This change in metabolism enables cancer cells to gather the components they require for growth and division, but it also leaves them open to treatments that aim to correct their altered metabolic state.

Recognizing the delicate balance our bodies must maintain to stay healthy is just as important as understanding biochemistry when it comes to understanding metabolism in the context of health and disease. It's about seeing how disease can result from a disruption in this equilibrium. Most importantly, it's about figuring out where we may possibly intervene to correct or lessen these disturbances, utilizing things like food, exercise, and even medication to help the body return to a state of metabolic balance.

How Cancer Cells Metabolize: The Warburg Effect

The Warburg effect, named after the Nobel laureate Otto Heinrich Warburg who first observed it, is a phenomenon where cancer cells predominantly produce energy by a high rate of glycolysis followed by lactic acid fermentation in the cytosol. This occurs even in the presence of sufficient oxygen, which would normally be utilized by healthy cells for more efficient energy production through oxidative phosphorylation in the mitochondria.

Warburg hypothesized that this metabolic shift towards what is essentially an inefficient means of energy production was a fundamental cause of cancer. This shift allows cancer cells to grow and proliferate even in environments where oxygen levels are too low for oxidative phosphorylation, which is the situation often found in rapidly growing tumors. The Warburg effect is characterized by an increased intake of glucose by cancer cells, a trait that has been exploited diagnostically with PET scans, where injected radioactive glucose analogs accumulate in cancerous tissues at higher concentrations than in normal tissues.

The underlying reasons for the Warburg effect are complex and multifaceted. One explanation is that the damage to mitochondria in cancer cells leads to a reliance on glycolysis for ATP production. Another is that cancer cells may deliberately reduce their mitochondrial activity as a way to evade apoptosis, the programmed cell death that is often initiated by mitochondrial signals.

The metabolic reprogramming of cancer cells is not just a means to generate energy; it also redirects resources towards the biosynthesis of nucleotides, amino acids, and lipids necessary for the creation of new cells. This is particularly advantageous for cancer cells as they need to proliferate rapidly. The Warburg effect, therefore, supports both the energy demands and the biosynthetic requirements of cancer cells.

Despite the initial belief that the Warburg effect was the cause of cancer, it is now understood that mutations in oncogenes and tumor suppressor genes are the primary drivers of malignant transformation. The Warburg effect is seen as a downstream consequence of these genetic changes. However, it remains a hallmark of cancer metabolism and a potential target for therapy.

The therapeutic implications of the Warburg effect have been a subject of research, with scientists exploring ways to target the altered metabolic pathways of cancer cells. Various substances that inhibit glycolysis have been developed with the potential to act as anticancer agents. However, the clinical efficacy of these substances is still under investigation, and there is no definitive evidence yet to support their use in cancer treatment.

CHAPTER 2

NUTRITIONAL SCIENCE FOR WOMEN

Macronutrients and Micronutrients: What Women Need

Macronutrients

Carbohydrates: These are the body's main energy source. Women should focus on consuming high-quality, fiber-rich carbohydrates such as fruits, vegetables, legumes, and whole grains. These complex carbohydrates provide a steady release of energy, which is essential for maintaining blood sugar levels and supporting overall hormonal balance.

The fiber in these foods also supports digestive health, which is crucial for proper nutrient absorption and can help in maintaining a healthy weight.

Proteins: These are the building blocks of life, essential for the repair and regeneration of tissues. Women require adequate protein intake to support muscle mass, which naturally declines with age.

Sources of high-quality protein include lean meats, poultry, fish, dairy products, eggs, legumes, and nuts.

These foods provide essential amino acids that the body cannot produce on its own.

During certain life stages, such as pregnancy or breastfeeding, women's protein needs increase significantly to support fetal development and milk production.

Fats: These are essential for numerous bodily functions, including hormone production. Women should focus on healthy fats, particularly those rich in omega-3 fatty acids, such as fatty fish, flaxseeds, chia seeds, and walnuts.

These fats are crucial for cardiovascular health, reducing inflammation, and may help in the prevention of mood disorders.

It's also important to include monounsaturated fats found in olive oil, avocados, and certain nuts, which can help manage cholesterol levels and support overall heart health.

Micronutrients

Iron: It is a critical nutrient, especially for menstruating women. It's a key component of hemoglobin, which carries oxygen in the blood. Iron-deficiency anemia is common among women and can lead to fatigue, weakness, and compromised immune function.

Good sources of iron include red meat, poultry, fish, lentils, spinach, and iron-fortified cereals. Vitamin C-rich foods can enhance iron absorption when eaten in conjunction.

Calcium and Vitamin D: It is vital for bone health, and women are at a higher risk for osteoporosis than men, especially after menopause due to the decrease in estrogen levels. Dairy products, leafy greens, and fortified foods are good sources of calcium.

Vitamin D is essential for calcium absorption and bone health. It can be synthesized in the skin through sunlight exposure and is also found in fatty fish, fortified milk, and egg yolks. Many women may require supplementation to achieve adequate Vitamin D levels, especially in areas with limited sunlight.

Folate (Vitamin B9): It is particularly important for women of childbearing age as it is essential for fetal development and can help prevent neural tube defects. Leafy greens, legumes, nuts, and fortified grains are excellent sources of folate.

Since folate needs increase significantly during pregnancy, supplementation is often recommended to ensure adequate intake.

Other Essential Micronutrients

Vitamin B12: Necessary for nerve function and the production of DNA and red blood cells. It's found primarily in animal products, so vegetarians and vegans may need to seek fortified foods or supplements.

Magnesium: Plays a role in over 300 enzyme reactions in the body, including energy creation, muscle movement, and nervous system regulation. Nuts, seeds, whole grains, and leafy green vegetables are good sources.

Zinc: Important for immune function, wound healing, DNA synthesis, and cell division. Zinc is found in a variety of foods, including meat, shellfish, legumes, seeds, and nuts.

The Impact of Hormones on Women's Metabolism

Hormones and Metabolic Rate

The thyroid gland plays a pivotal role in regulating metabolic rate through the secretion of thyroid hormones.

These hormones, thyroxine (T4) and triiodothyronine (T3), accelerate cellular functions, impacting how quickly the body burns calories. Women are more susceptible to thyroid disorders, which can lead to variations in metabolic rate, affecting weight and energy levels. Hypothyroidism, for example, can slow metabolism, leading to weight gain and fatigue, while hyperthyroidism can have the opposite effect.

Estrogen and Metabolism

Estrogen, one of the primary female sex hormones, has a profound effect on metabolism. It helps regulate glucose and lipid metabolism and influences how the body responds to insulin, the hormone that controls blood sugar levels. Estrogen promotes the storage of fat for reproductive purposes, which is why women typically have higher body fat percentages than men. However, this fat distribution changes with menopause, as lower estrogen levels can lead to a shift in fat storage from the hips and thighs to the abdominal area, increasing the risk of metabolic syndrome and cardiovascular disease.

Progesterone and Appetite

Progesterone, another key hormone in women's reproductive health, can increase appetite and may lead to weight gain if not managed with a balanced diet and regular exercise. Progesterone levels rise in the second half of the menstrual cycle, which can explain premenstrual cravings and increased hunger. Understanding these patterns can help women plan their diets and manage their caloric intake more effectively.

Hormones, Stress, and Weight Management

Cortisol, the stress hormone, can also affect women's metabolism. Chronic stress leads to prolonged cortisol secretion, which has been linked to abdominal fat accumulation. This type of fat is metabolically active and can contribute to inflammation and insulin resistance, increasing the risk of diabetes and heart disease.

Insulin Sensitivity Throughout the Menstrual Cycle

Women may experience changes in insulin sensitivity throughout the menstrual cycle. Estrogen tends to enhance sensitivity, while progesterone can decrease it. This fluctuation can affect energy levels and how the body processes carbohydrates, making blood sugar management more challenging for women, especially those with conditions like Polycystic Ovary Syndrome (PCOS), which is characterized by insulin resistance.

The Role of Leptin and Ghrelin

Leptin and ghrelin, hormones involved in appetite regulation, also play a role in women's metabolism. Leptin, which signals satiety, tends to be higher in women than men, possibly due to higher body fat percentages. However, leptin resistance can develop, blunting this signal and leading to overeating. Ghrelin, which signals hunger, can be influenced by sleep patterns, which in turn can be affected by progesterone.

Hormonal Changes During Menopause

During menopause, the decrease in estrogen and progesterone levels can lead to a slower metabolism, making weight management more challenging. The loss of lean muscle mass with age (sarcopenia) further slows metabolism, emphasizing the need for strength training and protein-rich diets to maintain muscle mass and metabolic health.

Nutritional Strategies to Support Hormonal Balance

A diet rich in fiber, healthy fats, lean proteins, and complex carbohydrates can support hormonal balance. Phytoestrogens, found in foods like soy, can mimic the effects of estrogen and may be beneficial during menopause. Regular consumption of cruciferous vegetables like broccoli and Brussels sprouts can support liver function and hormonal balance due to their content of indole-3-carbinol.

CHAPTER 3

EXERCISE PHYSIOLOGY FOR CANCER PREVENTION

Exercise physiology is the study of the body's responses to physical activity and how these responses can be harnessed to prevent or manage diseases, including cancer. The premise here is that exercise affects our body at a molecular level, influencing everything from hormone levels to immune function. For cancer prevention, the physiological changes induced by regular physical activity can alter the environment within our bodies, making it less conducive for cancer to develop and progress.

How Physical Activity Influences Cellular Health

Physical activity is a cornerstone of preventive medicine. It exerts its effects on cellular health through various mechanisms:

1. Modulation of Inflammation:

Physical activity has been shown to reduce systemic inflammation, a chronic condition that can lead to DNA damage and subsequent cancer development. Exercise stimulates the production of anti-inflammatory cytokines while inhibiting the release of pro-inflammatory substances. This shift in the inflammatory balance is crucial because chronic inflammation can provide a supportive environment for the initiation and progression of various cancers.

2. Enhancement of Immune Function:

Exercise can act as an adjuvant to the immune system. It promotes the circulation of immune cells, such as natural killer cells and T-cells, which are integral to identifying and destroying cancer cells. Regular physical activity ensures that these cells are more vigilant and effective, potentially lowering the risk of cancer development and aiding in the suppression of tumor growth.

3. Hormonal Regulation:

Hormones like insulin and estrogen play significant roles in cell proliferation and cancer risk. Exercise can help regulate these hormones, reducing levels of circulating insulin and related growth factors, which have been implicated in the development of insulin-resistant conditions and some cancers. For women, managing estrogen levels is particularly important, as high levels have been associated with an increased risk of breast and endometrial cancers. Physical activity can modulate estrogen metabolism, leading to a more favorable balance and potentially reducing cancer risk.

4. Reduction of Oxidative Stress:

While acute exercise induces a temporary increase in reactive oxygen species (ROS), chronic physical activity enhances the body's antioxidant defense systems. This adaptive response to regular exercise can mitigate oxidative stress, which is known to cause cellular damage, including DNA mutations that can initiate cancer.

5. DNA Repair and Protection:

Physical activity has been linked to the upregulation of DNA repair enzymes, which correct potentially mutagenic and carcinogenic DNA lesions. Moreover, exercise has been associated with the preservation of telomere length. Telomeres, which protect the ends of chromosomes, tend to shorten with age, and their accelerated shortening is associated with increased cancer risk. By preserving telomere length, exercise may contribute to chromosomal stability and a reduced risk of cancer.

6. Metabolic Regulation:

Exercise improves metabolic efficiency and can induce changes in energy metabolism that may protect against cancer. Enhanced mitochondrial function and the shift toward oxidative metabolism in muscles can reduce the availability of energy substrates for proliferating cancer cells. Furthermore, exercise-induced improvements in insulin sensitivity can decrease the likelihood of metabolic conditions that are associated with increased cancer risk.

7. Circadian Rhythms:

Emerging research suggests that physical activity can influence circadian rhythms, which are known to play a role in cellular functions, including cell cycle regulation and DNA repair processes. Disruptions in circadian rhythms have been implicated in cancer development, and regular physical activity may help to synchronize these rhythms and promote healthy cellular function.

8. Stress Response:

Exercise stimulates the production of stress proteins, which can protect cells from various types of damage. These proteins, including heat shock proteins, can prevent the aggregation of damaged proteins and assist in their repair or removal. This protective mechanism is vital for maintaining cellular integrity and preventing the accumulation of damage that could lead to cancer.

Tailoring Exercise to Women's Physiological Needs

It's clear that the manipulation of carbohydrate intake around exercise sessions can modulate cellular adaptations in skeletal muscle. This is relevant to cancer prevention as it underscores the importance of metabolic flexibility and the body's ability to efficiently switch between fuel sources, which can influence cellular health and potentially reduce cancer risk.

The concept of 'training low', This involves deliberately training with reduced carbohydrate availability to enhance metabolic adaptations. This approach has been shown to augment cell signaling, gene expression, and oxidative enzyme activity in muscle tissue. These adaptations are crucial because they can improve the muscle's ability to utilize oxygen and produce energy more efficiently, which is beneficial for overall health and may contribute to cancer prevention.

Women's hormonal fluctuations, bone density concerns, and specific risks for certain cancers, such as breast cancer, necessitate a nuanced approach to exercise prescription. For instance, understanding the glycogen cost of different types of exercise can help in designing training programs that optimize metabolic health without compromising energy levels or bone density.

To expand on the subheading "Tailoring Exercise to Women's Physiological Needs," we would need to consider several factors:

- **Menstrual Cycle Considerations:** Women's hormonal fluctuations throughout the menstrual cycle affect energy levels and metabolism. Exercise programs can be designed to align with these fluctuations, emphasizing different types of training at different points in the cycle to optimize performance and health outcomes.

- **Menopause and Metabolism:** As women approach menopause, changes in hormone levels can affect body composition and metabolic health. Tailored exercise programs can help mitigate these effects by focusing on resistance training to maintain muscle mass and metabolic rate.

- **Pregnancy and Postpartum:** For women who are pregnant or postpartum, exercise recommendations must be adapted to support the health of both mother and child, with a focus on moderate-intensity activities and exercises that strengthen the core and pelvic floor.

- **Breast Cancer Survivors:** For women who are breast cancer survivors, exercise programs should be designed to improve lymphatic function, manage fatigue, and support overall well-being, often incorporating a mix of aerobic, resistance, and flexibility training.

- **Bone Health:** Women are at a higher risk for osteoporosis, so weight-bearing and resistance exercises are essential to maintain bone density and prevent fractures.

- **Psychosocial Support:** Exercise programs for women should also consider the importance of social support, body image, and community, as these factors can significantly influence motivation and adherence to a healthy lifestyle.

CHAPTER 4

ANTI-CANCER FOODS FOR WOMEN

The concept of anti-cancer foods stems from the understanding that certain dietary components can support the body's natural defenses against cancer development. For women, this is particularly important due to the unique risk factors they face, such as breast and ovarian cancers. The foods we eat can influence a variety of bodily processes, including hormone levels, inflammation, and immune function, all of which play roles in cancer risk.

A diet rich in certain foods can provide a powerful blend of nutrients that work synergistically to protect cells from damage, inhibit the growth of cancer cells, and boost overall health. These foods are typically high in vitamins, minerals, fiber, and a host of phytochemicals and antioxidants that have been shown to possess anti-cancer properties.

Phytochemicals and Antioxidants: A Woman's Armor

Phytochemicals are compounds produced by plants that have various health benefits. They are not essential nutrients like vitamins and minerals, but they can influence the chemical processes inside our bodies in a way that could reduce the risk of certain diseases. For women, phytochemicals can be particularly potent in the fight against cancer. They work in several ways, such as detoxifying carcinogens, slowing the growth of cancer cells, and being potent antioxidants.

Antioxidants are substances that can prevent or slow damage to cells caused by free radicals, which are unstable molecules that the body produces as a response to environmental and other pressures. For women, antioxidants can be considered as armor against cancer because they protect cells from damage that could lead to cancer development.

Some key phytochemicals and antioxidants include:

Flavonoids: Found in fruits, vegetables, and certain beverages like tea and red wine, flavonoids have been linked to a lower risk of cancer.

Carotenoids: These are the pigments that give fruits and vegetables like carrots, sweet potatoes, and spinach their vibrant colors. Beta-carotene, lycopene, and lutein are types of carotenoids that have antioxidant properties.

Sulforaphane: Found in cruciferous vegetables like broccoli, Brussels sprouts, and kale, sulforaphane has been shown to have anti-cancer effects.

Lignans: Found in high fiber foods such as flaxseeds, sesame seeds, and whole grains, lignans have antioxidant properties and may influence hormone metabolism in ways that could deter cancer.

Incorporating a variety of these phytochemicals and antioxidants into a woman's diet can help form a protective barrier against cancer. It's not about single "superfoods" but rather a diverse diet rich in these compounds.

Superfoods in the Fight Against Cancer

The term "superfoods" has captured the public's imagination and is often used to describe foods that are thought to have health benefits beyond their nutritional value. In the context of cancer, these foods are lauded for their high concentrations of critical nutrients and compounds that may help prevent the onset or progression of cancer. Here's a closer look at some of these superfoods:

- **Berries**: Berries are a powerhouse of vitamins, minerals, fiber, and particularly high levels of antioxidants such as vitamin C and flavonoids. The antioxidants in berries can help fight oxidative stress and reduce inflammation, which are both linked to cancer. For example, the anthocyanins, which give berries their red, blue, and purple hues, have been shown in studies to inhibit tumor growth and spread.

- **Leafy Greens:** Leafy green vegetables like spinach, kale, and collard greens are rich in vitamins, minerals, and fiber. They contain high levels of carotenoids, which studies suggest can inhibit the growth of certain types of breast, skin, lung, and stomach cancer. They also have folate, which plays a role in DNA repair and synthesis and may reduce the risk of cancer caused by DNA mutations.

- **Nuts and Seeds:** Nuts and seeds are good sources of protein, healthy fats, and fiber. They also contain various vitamins and minerals, as well as antioxidants and phytochemicals. For instance, flaxseeds contain lignans, which have been found to slow the growth of tumor cells in several types of cancer. Walnuts are rich in omega-3 fatty acids, which may help reduce inflammation and the potential for breast and prostate cancer.

- **Legumes:** Beans, lentils, and peas are not only high in fiber but also contain a variety of cancer-fighting phytochemicals. Fiber itself is known to help reduce the risk of colorectal cancer. Legumes also have saponins, protease inhibitors, and phytic acid, which are thought to protect cells from the DNA damage that can lead to cancer.

- **Cruciferous Vegetables:** This group of vegetables, which includes broccoli, cauliflower, Brussels sprouts, and cabbage, contains glucosinolates, which are chemicals that produce protective enzymes when broken down. Sulforaphane, derived from glucosinolates, has been shown to have potent anti-cancer properties in laboratory studies, including the potential to induce cell death in cancer cells.

- **Garlic and Onions:** These vegetables belong to the allium family and are rich in compounds like allicin, which has been shown to have anti-cancer properties. Studies have linked the consumption of garlic and onions to a reduced risk of stomach and colorectal cancers, possibly due to their ability to inhibit the growth of cancer cells and induce apoptosis (cell death).

- **Turmeric:** The compound curcumin, found in turmeric, is one of the most extensively studied for its anti-cancer properties. It has been shown to interfere with multiple cell signaling pathways and inhibit the transformation, proliferation, and invasion of cancerous cells. Curcumin also has potent anti-inflammatory and antioxidant effects, which may contribute to its potential anti-cancer effects.

- **Green Tea:** Rich in polyphenols, especially catechins, green tea is another superfood with anti-cancer potential. Epigallocatechin-3-gallate (EGCG) is the most studied catechin in green tea and has been shown to inhibit the growth of cancer cells and prevent the spread of tumors.

- **Whole Grains:** Whole grains contain fiber, vitamins, minerals, and a variety of phytochemicals that may collectively contribute to cancer prevention. The fiber in whole grains not only helps with digestive health but may also reduce the risk of colorectal cancer. Additionally, certain phytochemicals found in whole grains, such as saponins and lignans, have been shown to have anti-cancer effects.

- **Tomatoes:** Rich in lycopene, tomatoes have been studied for their potential role in cancer prevention, particularly prostate cancer. Lycopene is a potent antioxidant that may help prevent cancer by neutralizing harmful free radicals that can damage cells and DNA.

CHAPTER 5

DIETARY PATTERNS FOR METABOLIC HEALTH

The Mediterranean Diet and Cancer Prevention

The MD is not just a diet; it's a tapestry of cultural and culinary practices that have been honed over centuries in the Mediterranean basin. At its core, it emphasizes the consumption of a variety of plant-based foods: fruits, vegetables, whole grains, legumes, and nuts. These are the unsung heroes of the diet, providing a bounty of fibers, vitamins, minerals, and a plethora of phytochemicals that have been shown to have anti-carcinogenic properties.

Olive oil is the maestro of this symphony, orchestrating a healthier fat intake with its monounsaturated fats and polyphenols like oleocanthal, which have been studied for their anti-inflammatory and potential cancer-inhibiting effects. The diet's modest portion of dairy, primarily in the form of cheese and yogurt, adds a fermentative dimension, introducing beneficial probiotics and additional nutrients.

Seafood, a staple protein source in the MD, brings in omega-3 fatty acids, known for their anti-inflammatory effects. The diet's low consumption of red meat is a strategic move to minimize the intake of saturated fats and heme iron, which have been associated with increased cancer risk in numerous studies.

Red Wine: A Controversial Companion

Red wine, when consumed in moderation, is a part of the MD and is valued for its polyphenols, such as resveratrol. These compounds have been the subject of intense research due to their potential to modulate several cancer-related processes. However, the relationship between alcohol and cancer is complex, and moderation is key. The protective effects of wine's polyphenols must be balanced against the risks associated with alcohol consumption.

Scientific Insights: The MD and Cancer Prevention

A plethora of studies have illuminated the MD's potential in cancer prevention. The diet's high fiber content is particularly beneficial for gastrointestinal health, with a robust inverse correlation between fiber intake and colorectal cancer risk. The antioxidants present in the diet's fruits and vegetables, such as vitamin C, lycopene, and beta-carotene, contribute to a cellular defense system that combats oxidative damage—a precursor to cancer.

The anti-inflammatory profile of the MD is another cornerstone of its cancer-fighting reputation. Chronic inflammation is a recognized accomplice in the development of cancer, and the MD's rich supply of anti-inflammatory nutrients can disrupt this insidious process. The diet's ability to influence weight management also plays a role, as obesity is a well-established risk factor for several cancers.

Evidence in Practice: Adherence and Outcomes

Epidemiological evidence suggests that adherence to the MD correlates with a lower incidence of various cancers. For instance, breast cancer, which has a known hormonal component, appears to be less prevalent among those who follow the MD, potentially due to the diet's influence on hormone levels and metabolism.

The inverse relationship extends to other cancers as well, including gastric and lung cancer. The mechanisms are multifaceted, involving the diet's impact on body weight,

44

inflammation, and even genetic expression related to cell proliferation and apoptosis (programmed cell death).

Beyond Prevention: The MD in Cancer Survivorship

The MD's role extends into the realm of cancer survivorship, where it may help mitigate the risk of recurrence and promote a better quality of life. The diet's nutrient-dense profile supports the body's recovery during and after cancer treatment, providing the energy and building blocks necessary for healing.

A Holistic Approach: The MD as Part of a Lifestyle

The MD is more than a collection of foods; it's a lifestyle. Physical activity, social engagement, and a general emphasis on enjoying meals slowly and in the company of others are integral to the Mediterranean way of life. These factors contribute to the overall health benefits observed and are essential components of a cancer-preventive lifestyle.

Relationship Between Weight Loss and Cancer in Women

Cancer as a Cause of Weight Loss: Cancer can sometimes lead to unexplained weight loss in women. This unintentional weight loss may be a symptom of an underlying cancer, particularly in advanced stages. Certain cancers, such as pancreatic, stomach, and esophageal cancers, are more likely to cause weight loss due to their impact on the digestive system and metabolism.

Cancer Treatment and Weight Changes: The treatment for cancer, including chemotherapy and radiation therapy, can also lead to weight changes. Some cancer treatments may cause weight gain, while others can result in weight loss due to side effects like nausea, loss of appetite, and metabolic changes. This can affect a woman's body weight during and after cancer treatment.

Obesity and Cancer Risk: On the other hand, being overweight or obese is a well-established risk factor for several types of cancer, including breast, uterine, ovarian, and colorectal cancers. Excess body fat can promote the development of cancer by causing chronic inflammation and hormonal imbalances in the body.

Weight Management and Cancer Prevention: Maintaining a healthy weight through proper diet and regular physical activity is an important factor in cancer prevention for women. A balanced lifestyle can reduce the risk of developing obesity-related cancers.

Nutrition and Cancer: A nutritious diet is crucial in both cancer prevention and treatment. Eating a variety of fruits, vegetables, whole grains, and lean proteins can help support the body's immune system and overall health. Nutrient-rich foods can also be important for women undergoing cancer treatment to maintain their strength and manage treatment side effects.

Physical Activity and Cancer Risk: Regular physical activity is associated with a lower risk of certain cancers. Exercise helps control body weight, improve overall health, and reduce the risk of developing obesity-related cancers. It can also help women with cancer cope with the physical and emotional challenges of their diagnosis and treatment.

Pros of the Ketogenic Diet for Women's Health

Weight Loss: Many women report short-term weight loss on the keto diet due to its high-fat, low-carbohydrate regimen. The diet's structure can lead to a decrease in appetite and an increase in satiety, which may help reduce overall calorie intake.

Metabolic Impact: By significantly reducing carbohydrate intake, the keto diet forces the body to burn fat for fuel in a state known as ketosis. This metabolic state can be particularly beneficial for women with metabolic disorders, including type 2 diabetes and obesity.

Nutritional Awareness: The restrictive nature of the keto diet often leads to increased awareness of food and nutrient intake. This can encourage the adoption of healthier eating habits, such as choosing nutrient-dense foods and cooking at home.

Neurological Benefits: Preliminary research suggests that the keto diet may offer benefits for neurological health. While traditionally used to reduce seizures in epilepsy, there is ongoing research into its effects on other neurological conditions.

Cons of the Ketogenic Diet for Women's Health

Nutrient Deficiencies: The keto diet's strict limits on carbohydrates can lead to deficiencies in essential vitamins and minerals, particularly vitamin A, C, K, folate, and dietary fiber. This can be a significant concern for women's long-term health.

Keto Flu: The transition to ketosis can be accompanied by symptoms such as headaches, fatigue, and nausea, often referred to as the "keto flu." These symptoms can be particularly challenging for women to manage alongside their daily responsibilities.

Heart Health Risks: High intake of saturated fats, which can be common in a poorly planned keto diet, may increase the risk of cardiovascular diseases. Women need to be cautious about the types of fats they consume while on the keto diet.

Sustainability Issues: The keto diet is highly restrictive, making it difficult to sustain long-term. This can lead to a pattern of "yo-yo dieting," which has been associated with negative health outcomes and increased mortality.

Impact on Kidney Health: The increased production of ketones and the potential for a high intake of protein can put additional strain on the kidneys. Women with pre-existing kidney conditions need to be particularly cautious.

Psychological Effects: The intensive monitoring of food intake required by the keto diet can lead to an unhealthy obsession with food and may contribute to psychological distress, disordered eating patterns, or eating disorders.

Bone Health Concerns: There is some evidence to suggest that the keto diet may affect bone health due to changes in acid-base balance and potential calcium losses, which is a crucial consideration for women, particularly as they age.

Reproductive Health: The impact of the keto diet on women's reproductive health is not fully understood, but there are concerns that the diet could affect menstrual regularity and fertility due to its potential impact on hormones.

CHAPTER 6

SUPPLEMENTS AND WOMEN'S HEALTH

Vitamins and Mineral Supplements for Women's Health Against Cancer

Vitamin D: This vitamin is crucial for bone health and has been linked to a lower risk of certain cancers, including breast cancer. Vitamin D may play a role in regulating cell growth and supporting immune function. However, it's essential to monitor levels and consult with a healthcare provider to avoid excessive intake, which could be harmful.

Folate (Vitamin B9): Adequate folate is essential for DNA synthesis and repair. A deficiency may increase the risk of cancer development. However, there is a delicate balance as high levels of synthetic folic acid from supplements have been associated with increased cancer risk.

Antioxidants (Vitamins A, C, E): Antioxidants can protect cells from damage. However, there is controversy regarding their use during cancer treatment, as they may interfere with the effectiveness of radiation therapy and certain chemotherapies by protecting cancer cells from oxidative damage.

Calcium: Important for bone health, especially in postmenopausal women, calcium may also have a role in protecting against colorectal cancer. However, excessive calcium intake has been linked to an increased risk of prostate cancer in men and may have unknown effects in women.

Selenium: This mineral has antioxidant properties and may help protect against cancer. Some studies suggest a lower cancer risk with adequate selenium intake, but the evidence is not conclusive, and high doses can be toxic.

Iron: Iron is essential for transporting oxygen in the blood, but excess iron can lead to oxidative stress and has been linked to an increased risk of colorectal and possibly other cancers. Iron supplementation should be based on individual needs and blood levels.

Zinc: Zinc is vital for immune function and DNA repair. While a deficiency can impair these processes and potentially increase cancer risk, excessive zinc intake can also have negative effects.

Omega-3 Fatty Acids: While not a vitamin or mineral, omega-3 supplements are often considered for their anti-inflammatory properties and potential to reduce the risk of breast cancer. However, the evidence is mixed, and they should be used cautiously.

Risks and Considerations of Vitamin and Mineral Supplements

Supplement Quality: The quality and purity of supplements can vary, and some may contain contaminants or not contain the labeled amounts of vitamins or minerals.

Interactions with Treatment: Some supplements can interfere with cancer treatments, either by reducing their effectiveness or by increasing side effects.

Hormone-Sensitive Cancers: Supplements that affect hormone levels, such as some herbal supplements, should be used with caution, especially in hormone-sensitive cancers like breast cancer.

Dosage: The appropriate dose of vitamins and minerals can vary widely based on individual health status, dietary intake, and specific health conditions.

Medical Supervision: It's crucial for women, especially those with cancer or at high risk for cancer, to discuss any supplements with their healthcare provider to ensure they are safe and appropriate.

Herbs for Women Health Against Cancer

Herbs have been used for centuries in various cultures for their medicinal properties, and modern research has begun to explore their potential benefits in the context of cancer prevention and treatment. Here is a comprehensive list and explanation of herbs that may be beneficial for women's health against cancer, based on the synthesized information from the sources provided:

- **Ginger:** Containing a compound called 6-shogaol, ginger has been found to be effective at killing cancer cells while sparing healthy cells. It's also beneficial for the immune system and gut health, which are crucial for cancer recovery. Ginger can be consumed as tea or used in cooking.

- **Aloe Vera:** Known for its soothing properties, aloe vera also contains polysaccharides that boost the immune system and may help destroy cancer cells. It can be consumed as juice or used topically, particularly for skin cancers.

- **Rosemary:** This herb contains carnosic acid and carnosol, which are potent cancer-fighting agents. Rosemary also helps protect the body against radiation exposure and supports brain health. It can be added to meals or used to make tea.

- **Garlic:** Garlic's sulfur compounds have been shown to neutralize carcinogens and contribute to tumor shrinkage. It is considered one of nature's best remedies for various health issues, including cancer.

- **Turmeric:** With curcumin as its active component, turmeric is a powerful tumor destroyer and immune system booster. It's recommended to be taken with black pepper and a fat source like coconut oil to enhance absorption.

- **Red Clover:** Used in traditional medicine, red clover contains anti-tumor compounds and a strong antioxidant, tocopherol. It's been used globally as a first-line treatment for cancer.

- **Astragalus:** Research has indicated that astragalus can double the survival rate of cancer patients compared to a placebo. It's recognized for its effectiveness across various types of cancer.

- **Cat's Claw:** This vine from the Peruvian jungle boosts the immune system and is known for its cancer-fighting properties. It increases the production of T-cells, which attack and destroy cancer cells.

- **Essiac Tea:** A traditional Native American remedy, Essiac Tea has been used as a cancer treatment for decades. It's a blend of herbs known to have anti-cancer properties.

- **Turmeric (Curcumin):** Curcumin, the active ingredient in turmeric, is a potent anti-inflammatory that may help prevent cancer by counteracting the blood vessels that feed cancer cells.

- **Black Pepper:** Found to inhibit the growth of cancerous stem cells, especially when combined with turmeric.

- **Cayenne Pepper:** Contains capsaicin, which may stifle the growth of cancer cells and in some cases, kill them.

- **Allspice:** Known for its anti-inflammatory properties, allspice is often used in various cuisines and has potential cancer-fighting benefits.

- **Oregano:** Contains carvacrol, which may help offset the spread of cancer cells by acting as a natural disinfectant.

- **Saffron:** Contains crocins that may inhibit tumor growth and progression.

- **Thyme:** Similar to oregano, thyme contains carvacrol and has potential anti-cancer properties.

- **Lavender:** Some studies have identified compounds in lavender that may be helpful against cancer.

CHAPTER 7

BUILDING A CANCER-RESISTANT BODY

The pursuit of a cancer-resistant body is a multifaceted endeavor that involves more than just avoiding carcinogens. It's about creating an internal environment where cancer cells are less likely to thrive. This involves a combination of proper nutrition, regular exercise, stress management, and adequate sleep. Among the pillars of this approach, exercise stands out for its dual role in prevention and as a supportive therapy for those undergoing cancer treatment.

Strength Training: The Unsung Heroine

Strength training, often overshadowed by the more publicized cardiovascular exercises, is a critical component of building a cancer-resistant body. It goes beyond aesthetic benefits, playing a significant role in enhancing metabolic health, which can be particularly protective against cancer.

- **The Biological Impact:** Muscle tissue is metabolically active, meaning it consumes calories even at rest. By increasing lean muscle mass through strength training, the body's resting metabolic rate (RMR) increases, which can help in maintaining a healthy body weight – a key factor in cancer prevention. Obesity has been linked to an increased risk of several cancers, including breast, colon, and endometrial cancers.

- Moreover, strength training can help regulate blood sugar levels by improving insulin sensitivity. This is crucial because high insulin levels and insulin resistance are associated with an increased risk of cancer. Muscles that are engaged in regular strength training are better at absorbing glucose from the blood, which can lower blood sugar levels and potentially reduce cancer risk.

- **Hormonal Effects:** Strength training can also influence hormone levels in the body. For women, particularly, maintaining a balanced level of hormones like estrogen is essential, as high levels have been associated with an increased risk of breast and ovarian cancers. Regular strength training has been shown to help balance hormone levels, which could contribute to a lower risk of hormone-related cancers.

- **Immune System Enhancement:** Physical activity, including strength training, can boost the immune system. It can lead to an increase in the circulation of immune cells in the body, which are critical in identifying and destroying cancer cells. The transient increase in body temperature during exercise may also play a role in inhibiting the growth of cancer cells.

- **Psychological Benefits:** The psychological benefits of strength training are also noteworthy. It has been linked to reduced anxiety, depression, and fatigue, all of which can be particularly beneficial for those at risk of cancer or undergoing treatment. The sense of empowerment and control that comes with strength training can also improve the overall quality of life and well-being.

Cardiovascular Health: More Than Heart Deep

While strength training is crucial, cardiovascular health cannot be overlooked. Cardiovascular exercise, also known as aerobic exercise, includes activities like walking, running, cycling, and swimming. These exercises increase the heart rate and improve the efficiency of the cardiovascular system.

- **Oxygen and Nutrient Delivery:** Improved cardiovascular health enhances the delivery of oxygen and nutrients to all tissues in the body, including those that are part of the immune system. This enhanced circulation can support the body's natural defense mechanisms against cancer.

- **Inflammation Reduction:** Chronic inflammation is a known risk factor for cancer. Cardiovascular exercise can lead to reductions in inflammatory markers in the body. Regular aerobic exercise has been shown to lower levels of certain inflammatory substances, which could potentially reduce the risk of cancer.

- **Body Weight Management:** Cardiovascular exercise is effective in burning calories and is thus a cornerstone of weight management strategies. As mentioned earlier, maintaining a healthy weight is important in reducing cancer risk.

- **Detoxification:** By increasing blood flow and lymphatic circulation, cardiovascular exercise can help in the detoxification process. The lymphatic system, which is stimulated by muscle movement, plays a role in removing waste and toxins from the body.

- **Stress Hormone Regulation:** Exercise is a well-known stress reliever. It can reduce levels of the body's stress hormones, such as adrenaline and cortisol. High levels of these hormones can suppress the immune system and have been associated with increased cancer risk.

Yoga and Mind-Body Wellness

Yoga is an ancient practice with a rich history spanning over 3,000 years, traditionally aimed at unifying the body and mind to achieve a state of harmony and balance. In contemporary times, yoga is recognized not just as a physical exercise but as a holistic mind-body fitness regimen that integrates physical postures, breathing exercises, and meditation. The essence of yoga lies in its ability to foster an internal environment of mindfulness, where the practitioner's attention is directed towards the self, breath, and energy, creating a physiological state that counters the stress response.

The Role of Stress Reduction in Cancer Prevention

- Stress has been identified as a contributing factor to the etiology of numerous diseases, including heart disease, cancer, and stroke. The mechanism through which stress affects the body is complex, involving a cascade of hormonal and physiological responses that can lead to a state of chronic inflammation and reduced immune function, both of which are known to contribute to the development and progression of cancer.

- Yoga, as a holistic stress management technique, has been shown to produce a physiological sequence of events in the body that reduces the stress response. This is achieved through the practice of asanas (body postures) and pranayama (breathing techniques), which together help to shift the balance from the sympathetic nervous system (responsible for the fight-or-flight response) to the parasympathetic nervous system (which promotes the relaxation response). The relaxation response is calming and restorative, lowering breathing and heart rates, decreasing blood pressure, reducing cortisol levels, and increasing blood flow to vital organs.

- In the context of cancer prevention, the reduction of stress is paramount. Chronic stress can lead to hormonal imbalances and immune suppression, making the body more susceptible to cellular mutations and the proliferation of cancer cells. By incorporating yoga into one's lifestyle, an individual can enhance their body's resilience against stress and, consequently, against the factors that contribute to cancer development.

Yoga: Harmonizing Body and Mind

- The practice of yoga is not merely a series of physical exercises; it is a discipline that encompasses the health of the entire individual—physical, mental, and spiritual. The philosophy of yoga, as described by Patanjali in the classic text "Yoga Sutras," outlines an eightfold path known as ashtanga, which includes ethical principles, self-discipline, and spiritual enlightenment. These principles guide the practitioner towards a harmonious state where the health of the body is inextricably linked to the tranquility of the mind.

- Yoga's approach to harmonizing the body and mind involves a deep understanding that the human body is a holistic entity comprised of interrelated dimensions. The health or illness of any one dimension affects the others. This understanding is crucial in the treatment and prevention of disease, as it acknowledges the individuality of each person and tailors the yogic practice to their unique needs.

- Through sustained practice, yoga promotes strength, endurance, flexibility, and cultivates qualities such as friendliness, compassion, and self-control. It also fosters a sense of well-being, relaxation, and improved self-confidence. These outcomes are not just beneficial for physical health but are essential for mental health, providing a sense of energy and enjoyment in life.

- In the therapeutic context, yoga is used to alleviate structural, physiological, emotional, and spiritual pain and limitations. It has been found to enhance muscular strength, improve respiratory and cardiovascular function, aid in the recovery from addiction, reduce stress, anxiety, depression, and chronic pain, improve sleep patterns, and enhance overall well-being and quality of life.

- The practice of Hatha yoga, one of the most common forms of yoga in the Western world, emphasizes the unification of the physical body with breath and concentration. This unification clears blockages in the energy channels of the body and balances the body's energy system. The Iyengar method of Hatha yoga, in particular,

66

focuses on strength, stability, stamina, and body alignment, using props to facilitate learning and adjust poses to ease various ailments and stressors.

Creating Your Personalized Exercise Plan

This is a critical step towards achieving and maintaining optimal health, especially when considering the unique needs of women in the context of cancer prevention. The goal of such a plan is to tailor fitness activities to individual capabilities, health status, and personal objectives, ensuring that the regimen is both effective and sustainable over the long term. To construct a personalized exercise plan, it's essential to begin with an assessment of one's current fitness level and then to set realistic and sustainable goals. This approach not only helps in crafting a plan that is attuned to one's current health but also sets the stage for gradual and consistent progress.

Assessing Your Fitness Level

Before embarking on any new exercise routine, it's crucial to evaluate your starting point. This assessment should be comprehensive, covering cardiovascular fitness, muscular strength and endurance, flexibility, and body composition. Here's how you can assess each component:

- **Cardiovascular Fitness:** This can be gauged by how quickly your heart rate returns to normal after a period of physical activity. A simple way to test this is by taking a brisk walk or a light jog and timing your recovery after stopping.

- **Muscular Strength and Endurance:** To assess this, you can see how many push-ups, squats, or other bodyweight exercises you can perform before muscle fatigue sets in.

- **Flexibility:** This can be measured by the range of motion in your joints. For example, a sit-and-reach test can help determine the flexibility of your lower back and hamstring muscles.

- **Body Composition:** This refers to the proportion of fat versus lean muscle tissue in your body. While there are sophisticated methods to measure body composition, a simple start could be calculating your Body Mass Index (BMI) or using a tape measure to track waist circumference.

After assessing these areas, you'll have a clearer picture of your strengths and areas that may need more focus. It's also advisable to consult with a healthcare provider or a fitness professional to ensure that your self-assessment is accurate and to identify any potential health risks.

Setting Realistic and Sustainable Goals

Once you have a baseline of your fitness level, the next step is to set goals. Goals should be SMART: Specific, Measurable, Achievable, Relevant, and Time-bound.

Specific: Clearly define what you want to achieve. Instead of a vague goal like "get fit," aim for something more precise, such as "be able to jog 5 kilometers without stopping."

Measurable: Ensure that you can track your progress. If your goal is to improve strength, decide on how you'll measure that—perhaps by the number of repetitions of a certain exercise you can perform.

Achievable: Your goals should stretch your abilities but remain within reach. If you've never run before, setting a goal to complete a marathon in a month is unrealistic. A more achievable goal might be to run a 5K in three months.

Relevant: Your goals should be important to you and fit with your broader life objectives. If you're aiming to reduce cancer risk, your exercise goals should align with those that have been shown to have a positive impact on cancer prevention.

Time-bound: Set deadlines for your goals to give yourself a clear target to work towards. This helps with motivation and prioritization.

With these principles in mind, you can begin to outline your exercise plan. Here's an example of what that might look like:

Weeks 1-4: Foundation Building

Cardio: Walking 30 minutes, 5 days a week.

Strength: Bodyweight exercises twice a week.

Flexibility: Stretching routine daily.

Weeks 5-8: Intensity Increase

Cardio: Introduce jogging intervals into walks.

Strength: Add light weights or resistance bands.

Flexibility: Incorporate yoga once a week.

Weeks 9-12: Consistency and Growth

Cardio: Jog for 30 minutes, 4 days a week.

Strength: Increase weight or resistance level.

Flexibility: Attend two yoga classes per week.

Weeks 13-16: Goal Assessment and Adjustment

Re-evaluate fitness level.

Adjust goals based on progress.

Introduce new activities to keep the routine engaging.

Remember, the key to a successful exercise plan is flexibility and adaptability. Listen to your body, and don't be afraid to adjust your goals as needed. Regular check-ins on your progress are vital, and they can be incredibly motivating as you start to see the fruits of your labor.

CHAPTER 8

IMPLEMENTING A METABOLIC APPROACH VIA RECIPES AND MEAL PLANNING

Breakfast Recipes

1. Berry Almond Oatmeal

Ingredients:

1 cup rolled oats

2 cups almond milk

1/2 cup mixed berries (blueberries, raspberries, blackberries)

1 tablespoon chia seeds

1 tablespoon almond butter

A sprinkle of cinnamon

A drizzle of honey (optional)

Instructions:

Combine oats and almond milk in a pot and bring to a simmer.

Cook until oats are soft, then stir in chia seeds and cinnamon.

Serve topped with berries, a dollop of almond butter, and a drizzle of honey if desired.

Nutritional Information:

Rich in fiber, antioxidants, and omega-3 fatty acids, this breakfast supports digestive health and provides anti-inflammatory benefits.

2. Spinach and Mushroom Egg White Scramble

Ingredients:

1 cup egg whites

1 cup fresh spinach

1/2 cup sliced mushrooms

1/4 cup diced onions

1 clove garlic, minced

Salt and pepper to taste

1 teaspoon olive oil

Instructions:

Sauté onions, garlic, and mushrooms in olive oil until tender.

Add spinach and cook until wilted.

Pour in egg whites and scramble until cooked through.

Season with salt and pepper.

Nutritional Information:

High in protein and low in calories, this scramble is also packed with vitamins and minerals that support cellular health.

3. Greek Yogurt with Flaxseeds and Walnuts

Ingredients:

1 cup Greek yogurt

2 tablespoons ground flaxseeds

1/4 cup walnuts, chopped

1 tablespoon honey

A handful of your favorite berries

Instructions:

Spoon Greek yogurt into a bowl.

Top with ground flaxseeds, walnuts, and berries.

Drizzle with honey for a touch of sweetness.

Nutritional Information: This combination provides a good balance of protein, healthy fats, and antioxidants, all of which are beneficial for metabolic health and cancer prevention.

4. Avocado Toast with Poached Egg

Ingredients:

2 slices of whole-grain bread

1 ripe avocado

2 eggs

Salt and pepper to taste

A pinch of red pepper flakes (optional)

Instructions:

Toast the bread to your liking.

Mash the avocado and spread it on the toast.

Poach the eggs and place them on top of the avocado.

Season with salt, pepper, and red pepper flakes if desired.

Nutritional Information:

Avocado provides healthy fats and fiber, while the eggs offer high-quality protein and essential nutrients.

5. Quinoa Breakfast Bowl

Ingredients:

1/2 cup quinoa

1 cup water

1/4 cup sliced almonds

1/2 teaspoon cinnamon

1 apple, diced

A drizzle of maple syrup

Instructions:

Rinse quinoa under cold water and drain.

Combine quinoa and water in a pot and bring to a boil.

Reduce heat and simmer until quinoa is fluffy.

Stir in cinnamon and transfer to a bowl.

Top with almonds, diced apple, and a drizzle of maple syrup.

Nutritional Information:

Quinoa is a complete protein and is high in fiber, while almonds add healthy fats and apples provide fiber and vitamin C.

6. Spicy Scrambled Tofu

Ingredients:

1 block firm tofu, drained and crumbled

1/2 teaspoon turmeric

1/2 teaspoon cayenne pepper

1/2 teaspoon black salt (kala namak, for an eggy flavor)

1 tablespoon nutritional yeast

1/2 bell pepper, diced

1/4 cup red onion, diced

1 tablespoon olive oil

Fresh herbs for garnish (e.g., parsley, cilantro)

Instructions:

Heat olive oil in a pan over medium heat.

Add the bell pepper and onion, sautéing until softened.

Stir in the crumbled tofu and spices (turmeric, cayenne pepper, and black salt).

Cook for about 5-7 minutes, then sprinkle nutritional yeast over the mixture.

Serve hot, garnished with fresh herbs.

Nutritional Information:

Tofu is a great source of plant-based protein, and the spices add metabolism-boosting properties. Nutritional yeast provides B-vitamins, and the vegetables add fiber and essential nutrients.

7. Chia and Berry Parfait

Ingredients:

3 tablespoons chia seeds

3/4 cup unsweetened almond milk

1/2 teaspoon vanilla extract

1 cup mixed berries (strawberries, blueberries, raspberries)

1/4 cup granola (optional)

Instructions:

In a bowl, mix chia seeds with almond milk and vanilla extract. Let it sit for at least 20 minutes or overnight in the refrigerator until it achieves a pudding-like consistency.

Layer the chia pudding with berries in a glass or bowl.

Top with granola for added texture and serve.

Nutritional Information:

Chia seeds are rich in omega-3 fatty acids and fiber, which are beneficial for heart health and may have anti-cancer properties. Berries are high in antioxidants and vitamins.

8. Savory Oatmeal with Greens

Ingredients:

1/2 cup steel-cut oats

1 3/4 cups water or vegetable broth

1 cup kale or spinach, chopped

1/4 cup cherry tomatoes, halved

1/4 teaspoon garlic powder

Salt and pepper to taste

1 tablespoon pumpkin seeds

Instructions:

Cook the steel-cut oats in water or vegetable broth according to package instructions.

A few minutes before the oats are done, stir in the chopped greens, cherry tomatoes, and garlic powder.

Continue cooking until the greens are wilted and the oats are creamy.

Season with salt and pepper, and garnish with pumpkin seeds before serving.

Nutritional Information:

Oats are a heart-healthy whole grain, and the addition of greens and tomatoes provides vitamins, minerals, and antioxidants. Pumpkin seeds add a nice crunch and are a good source of zinc.

Lunch Recipes

1. Mediterranean Tuna and White Bean Salad

Ingredients:

1 can of tuna in water, drained

1 can of white beans, rinsed and drained

1 cup of cherry tomatoes, halved

1/2 red onion, thinly sliced

A handful of fresh basil leaves, chopped

2 tablespoons of extra virgin olive oil

1 tablespoon of lemon juice

Salt and pepper to taste

Instructions:

In a large bowl, combine the tuna, white beans, cherry tomatoes, and red onion.

In a small bowl, whisk together the olive oil, lemon juice, salt, and pepper.

Pour the dressing over the salad and toss gently to combine.

Garnish with fresh basil before serving.

Nutritional Information:

High in protein from the tuna and beans, rich in fiber, and packed with antioxidants from the tomatoes and olive oil.

2. Quinoa and Roasted Vegetable Bowl

Ingredients:

1 cup of quinoa, cooked

2 cups of mixed vegetables (e.g., bell peppers, zucchini, and eggplant), chopped

1 tablespoon of olive oil

1 teaspoon of smoked paprika

Salt and pepper to taste

A handful of arugula

1 tablespoon of balsamic vinegar

Instructions:

Preheat the oven to 400°F (200°C).

Toss the chopped vegetables with olive oil, smoked paprika, salt, and pepper.

Spread the vegetables on a baking sheet and roast for 20-25 minutes until tender.

Serve the roasted vegetables over a bed of quinoa and arugula.

Drizzle with balsamic vinegar before serving.

Nutritional Information:

Quinoa provides a complete protein source, while the vegetables offer vitamins, minerals, and fiber.

3. Spinach and Berry Salad with Walnuts

Ingredients:

3 cups of fresh spinach leaves

1 cup of mixed berries (strawberries, blueberries, raspberries)

1/2 cup of walnuts, toasted

1/4 cup of crumbled feta cheese

2 tablespoons of olive oil

1 tablespoon of apple cider vinegar

1 teaspoon of honey

Salt and pepper to taste

Instructions:

In a large bowl, combine the spinach, mixed berries, and toasted walnuts.

In a small bowl, whisk together the olive oil, apple cider vinegar, honey, salt, and pepper to create the dressing.

Toss the salad with the dressing and sprinkle with feta cheese before serving.

Nutritional Information:

Berries are high in antioxidants, spinach provides iron and folate, and walnuts offer healthy fats.

4. Grilled Chicken and Avocado Wrap

Ingredients:

1 grilled chicken breast, sliced

1 ripe avocado, sliced

1 whole wheat wrap

1/2 cup of mixed greens

1 tablespoon of Greek yogurt

1 teaspoon of Dijon mustard

Salt and pepper to taste

Instructions:

Lay the whole wheat wrap flat and spread the Greek yogurt and Dijon mustard over the surface.

Add the mixed greens, sliced chicken breast, and avocado.

Season with salt and pepper, then roll the wrap tightly.

Cut in half and serve.

Nutritional Information:

Chicken is a lean protein, avocado provides healthy monounsaturated fats, and the whole wheat wrap offers complex carbohydrates.

5. Broccoli and Chickpea Stir-Fry

Ingredients:

1 cup of chickpeas, cooked

2 cups of broccoli florets

1 tablespoon of sesame oil

2 cloves of garlic, minced

1 teaspoon of grated ginger

2 tablespoons of low-sodium soy sauce

1 teaspoon of honey

Sesame seeds for garnish

Instructions:

Heat the sesame oil in a pan over medium heat.

Add the garlic and ginger, sautéing until fragrant.

Add the broccoli and stir-fry for a few minutes until it begins to soften.

Add the chickpeas, soy sauce, and honey, and stir-fry for another 5-7 minutes.

Garnish with sesame seeds before serving.

Nutritional Information: Broccoli is rich in fiber and vitamin C, chickpeas are a good source of protein and fiber, and sesame seeds add a dose of healthy fats.

6. Smashed Chickpea and Avocado Lettuce Wraps

Ingredients:

1 can (15 oz) chickpeas, drained and rinsed

1 ripe avocado

Juice of 1 lemon

1/2 red onion, finely chopped

1/2 cup cherry tomatoes, quartered

1/4 cup chopped cilantro

Salt and pepper to taste

Butter lettuce leaves for wrapping

Instructions:

In a bowl, mash the chickpeas and avocado together until well combined but still chunky.

Stir in lemon juice, red onion, cherry tomatoes, and cilantro. Season with salt and pepper.

Spoon the mixture into lettuce leaves and serve as wraps.

Nutritional Information:

Chickpeas are a great source of protein and fiber, while avocados provide healthy fats. This meal is rich in vitamins and antioxidants.

7. Quinoa with Roasted Cauliflower and Broccoli

Ingredients:

1 cup quinoa, rinsed

2 cups water

2 cups cauliflower florets

2 cups broccoli florets

1 tablespoon olive oil

1 teaspoon turmeric

Salt and pepper to taste

1/4 cup slivered almonds, toasted

1/4 cup dried cranberries

Instructions:

Preheat the oven to 425°F (220°C).

Toss cauliflower and broccoli with olive oil, turmeric, salt, and pepper. Spread on a baking sheet and roast for 20-25 minutes.

While vegetables are roasting, bring quinoa and water to a boil in a saucepan. Reduce heat to low, cover, and simmer for 15 minutes.

Fluff the cooked quinoa with a fork and mix in the roasted vegetables, almonds, and dried cranberries.

Nutritional Information:

Quinoa is a complete protein, and both cauliflower and broccoli are high in fiber and cancer-fighting compounds. Almonds add crunch and healthy fats.

8. Mediterranean White Bean and Sorghum Salad

Ingredients:

1 cup sorghum, cooked

1 can (15 oz) white beans, drained and rinsed

1 cup cherry tomatoes, halved

1 cucumber, diced

1/2 cup pitted Kalamata olives, halved

1/4 cup feta cheese, crumbled

1/4 cup fresh parsley, chopped

2 tablespoons olive oil

1 tablespoon red wine vinegar

Salt and pepper to taste

Instructions:

In a large bowl, combine cooked sorghum, white beans, cherry tomatoes, cucumber, olives, and feta cheese.

In a small bowl, whisk together olive oil, red wine vinegar, salt, and pepper to create a dressing.

Pour the dressing over the salad and toss to combine. Garnish with fresh parsley.

Nutritional Information:

Sorghum is a gluten-free grain rich in antioxidants. White beans are an excellent source of protein and fiber, and the vegetables and olives provide additional nutrients and healthy fats.

Dinner Recipes

1. Quinoa and Kale Salad with Berries and Nuts

Ingredients:

1 cup quinoa, cooked and cooled

2 cups kale, chopped

1/2 cup mixed berries (blueberries, raspberries, strawberries)

1/4 cup chopped nuts (almonds, walnuts)

2 tablespoons olive oil

1 tablespoon balsamic vinegar

Salt and pepper to taste

Instructions:

In a large bowl, combine the cooked quinoa and chopped kale.

Add the mixed berries and chopped nuts to the bowl.

In a small bowl, whisk together olive oil, balsamic vinegar, salt, and pepper.

Pour the dressing over the salad and toss to combine.

Serve chilled or at room temperature.

Nutritional Information:

This salad is rich in antioxidants from the berries, healthy fats from the nuts, and fiber from the quinoa and kale. It's a light yet satisfying meal that supports metabolic health.

2. Grilled Chicken with Avocado-Tomato Salsa

Ingredients:

2 boneless, skinless chicken breasts

1 ripe avocado, diced

1 cup cherry tomatoes, halved

1/4 cup red onion, finely chopped

Juice of 1 lime

2 tablespoons cilantro, chopped

Salt and pepper to taste

Olive oil for grilling

Instructions:

Preheat the grill to medium-high heat and lightly oil the grate.

Season the chicken breasts with salt and pepper and grill for 6-7 minutes on each side or until fully cooked.

In a bowl, combine the diced avocado, cherry tomatoes, red onion, lime juice, and cilantro. Season with salt and pepper to taste.

Once the chicken is cooked, let it rest for a few minutes, then serve topped with the avocado-tomato salsa.

Nutritional Information:

The chicken provides a lean protein source, while the avocado offers healthy monounsaturated fats. The tomatoes are high in lycopene, an antioxidant linked to cancer prevention.

3. Baked Salmon with Steamed Broccoli and Quinoa

Ingredients:

2 salmon fillets

1 tablespoon olive oil

1 teaspoon lemon zest

2 cups broccoli florets

1 cup quinoa, cooked

Salt and pepper to taste

Instructions:

Preheat the oven to 375°F (190°C).

Place the salmon fillets on a baking sheet, drizzle with olive oil, and sprinkle with lemon zest, salt, and pepper.

Bake in the preheated oven for 12-15 minutes or until the salmon flakes easily with a fork.

Steam the broccoli florets until tender-crisp, about 5 minutes.

Serve the baked salmon with a side of steamed broccoli and cooked quinoa.

Nutritional Information:

Salmon is an excellent source of omega-3 fatty acids, which have been shown to reduce inflammation and potentially lower the risk of cancer. Broccoli contains sulforaphane, a compound with potent anti-cancer properties.

4. Lentil Soup with Spinach and Carrots

Ingredients:

1 cup lentils, rinsed

4 cups vegetable broth

1 cup spinach, chopped

1 cup carrots, diced

1 onion, chopped

2 cloves garlic, minced

1 teaspoon cumin

Salt and pepper to taste

Olive oil for sautéing

Instructions:

In a large pot, heat olive oil over medium heat and sauté the onions and garlic until translucent.

Add the carrots and cook for a few more minutes.

Pour in the vegetable broth and lentils, bring to a boil, then reduce heat and simmer until the lentils are tender, about 20 minutes.

Stir in the spinach and cumin, and continue to simmer for another 5 minutes. Season with salt and pepper.

Serve hot.

Nutritional Information:

Lentils are a great source of plant-based protein and fiber. Spinach is rich in vitamins and minerals, and it has been associated with cancer prevention due to its high levels of antioxidants.

5. Tofu Stir-Fry with Mixed Vegetables

Ingredients:

1 block firm tofu, pressed and cubed

2 cups mixed vegetables (bell peppers, snap peas, mushrooms)

2 tablespoons soy sauce

1 tablespoon sesame oil

1 teaspoon ginger, grated

1 clove garlic, minced

Brown rice or cauliflower rice for serving

Instructions:

Heat the sesame oil in a large pan or wok over medium-high heat.

Add the tofu cubes and stir-fry until golden brown on all sides.

Add the garlic and ginger and stir-fry for another minute.

Add the mixed vegetables and soy sauce, and stir-fry until the vegetables are tender-crisp.

Serve over brown rice or cauliflower rice.

Nutritional Information:

Tofu is a complete protein and a good source of isoflavones, which have been studied for their role in cancer prevention. The vegetables add fiber and a variety of vitamins and minerals.

Snacks Recipes

1. Crispy Kale and Nutritional Yeast Bites

Ingredients:

2 cups of kale leaves, stems removed

1 tablespoon olive oil

2 tablespoons nutritional yeast

1/2 teaspoon salt

1/4 teaspoon garlic powder

Instructions:

Preheat your oven to 350°F (175°C).

In a bowl, toss the kale with olive oil until evenly coated.

Sprinkle the nutritional yeast, salt, and garlic powder over the kale and toss again.

Spread the kale on a baking sheet in a single layer.

Bake for 10-15 minutes until the edges are slightly brown and the kale is crispy.

Nutritional Information:

Rich in vitamins A, C, K, and B-complex.

Contains antioxidants and minerals.

2. Mixed Berry Chia Delight

Ingredients:

1/2 cup mixed berries (fresh or frozen)

3 tablespoons chia seeds

1 cup unsweetened almond milk

1 tablespoon honey or maple syrup (optional)

Instructions: In a jar, combine the chia seeds and almond milk. Stir well.

Let the mixture sit for 5 minutes, then stir again to prevent clumping.

Cover the jar and refrigerate for at least 2 hours, or overnight.

Once set to a pudding-like consistency, top with mixed berries and a drizzle of honey or maple syrup if desired.

Nutritional Information:

High in omega-3 fatty acids, fiber, and protein.

Antioxidant-rich from berries.

3. Spicy Roasted Chickpea Crunch

Ingredients:

1 can (15 oz) chickpeas, drained and rinsed

1 tablespoon olive oil

1/2 teaspoon cumin

1/4 teaspoon chili powder

1/4 teaspoon paprika

1/4 teaspoon salt

Instructions:

Preheat your oven to 400°F (200°C).

Pat the chickpeas dry with paper towels and remove any loose skins.

Toss the chickpeas with olive oil and spices until evenly coated.

Spread the chickpeas on a baking sheet and roast for 20-30 minutes, shaking the pan occasionally, until crispy.

Nutritional Information:

Good source of plant-based protein and dietary fiber.

Contains iron and several B vitamins.

4. Savory Mushroom Jerky

Ingredients:

2 cups thinly sliced mushrooms

2 tablespoons soy sauce or tamari

1 tablespoon apple cider vinegar

1/2 teaspoon smoked paprika

1/4 teaspoon garlic powder

Instructions:

In a bowl, whisk together soy sauce, apple cider vinegar, smoked paprika, and garlic powder.

Add the mushroom slices to the marinade and let sit for at least 30 minutes.

Preheat your oven to the lowest setting or use a dehydrator.

Place the mushrooms on a baking sheet lined with parchment paper.

Dehydrate in the oven or dehydrator until they reach a jerky-like consistency, typically 4-6 hours in the oven or as per the dehydrator's instructions.

Nutritional Information:

Low in calories and a good source of protein.

Provides selenium and several other minerals.

5. Vibrant Green Pea Hummus

Ingredients:

2 cups green peas, cooked and cooled

2 tablespoons tahini

1 tablespoon lemon juice

1 garlic clove, minced

2 tablespoons olive oil

Salt to taste

Instructions:

In a food processor, combine the green peas, tahini, lemon juice, and minced garlic.

Process until smooth, gradually adding olive oil until the desired consistency is reached.

Season with salt to taste.

Serve with vegetable sticks or whole-grain crackers.

Nutritional Information: Rich in plant-based protein and dietary fiber.

Contains vitamins A and C, as well as iron and calcium.

6. Onion and Flaxseed Crackers

Ingredients: 1 cup ground flaxseeds

1/2 cup water

1/2 cup caramelized onions, finely chopped

1/2 teaspoon salt

1 teaspoon dried thyme

Instructions: Preheat your oven to 350°F (175°C).

In a bowl, mix the ground flaxseeds with water and let sit for 5 minutes to thicken.

Stir in the caramelized onions, salt, and thyme.

Spread the mixture thinly on a baking sheet lined with parchment paper.

Bake for 20-25 minutes until the edges are golden and the center is firm.

Break into cracker-sized pieces after cooling.

Nutritional Information:

High in omega-3 fatty acids and fiber.

Contains phytonutrients and antioxidants.

7. Antioxidant-Packed Berry Spinach Smoothie

Ingredients: 1 cup fresh spinach leaves

1 cup mixed berries (fresh or frozen)

1 ripe banana

1 cup unsweetened almond milk

1 tablespoon hemp seeds

Instructions: Combine the spinach, berries, banana, almond milk, and hemp seeds in a blender.

Blend on high speed until smooth and creamy.

Pour into a glass and enjoy immediately.

Nutritional Information: Loaded with antioxidants, vitamins, and minerals.

Provides a healthy dose of plant-based protein and omega-3 fatty acids.

8. Pumpkin Seed and Goji Berry Trail Mix

Ingredients:

1/2 cup raw pumpkin seeds

1/2 cup goji berries

1/4 cup dark chocolate chips

1/2 cup raw almonds

1/4 cup unsweetened coconut flakes

Instructions: In a bowl, combine the pumpkin seeds, goji berries, dark chocolate chips, almonds, and coconut flakes.

Toss until well mixed.

Store in an airtight container and enjoy as a snack.

Nutritional Information: Rich in zinc, antioxidants, and healthy fats.

Provides a good balance of protein, fiber

21-Days Meal Plan

Day 1:

Breakfast: Oatmeal topped with mixed berries and a sprinkle of chia seeds.

Snack 1: Crispy Kale and Nutritional Yeast Bites.

Lunch: Quinoa salad with mixed greens, cherry tomatoes, and avocado.

Snack 2: A handful of Onion and Flaxseed Crackers.

Dinner: Grilled salmon with steamed broccoli and a side of brown rice.

Day 2:

Breakfast: Greek yogurt with granola and sliced strawberries.

Snack 1: Berry Spinach Smoothie.

Lunch: Turkey and hummus wrap with spinach and shredded carrots.

Snack 2: Spicy Roasted Chickpea Crunch.

Dinner: Stir-fried tofu with mixed vegetables over quinoa.

Day 3:

Breakfast: Scrambled eggs with spinach and mushrooms.

Snack 1: A small bowl of Mixed Berry Chia Delight.

Lunch: Lentil soup with a side of whole-grain bread.

Snack 2: Pumpkin Seed and Goji Berry Trail Mix.

Dinner: Baked chicken breast with roasted sweet potatoes and green beans.

Day 4:

Breakfast: Smoothie with spinach, banana, almond milk, and a scoop of protein powder.

Snack 1: Vibrant Green Pea Hummus with vegetable sticks.

Lunch: Grilled chicken salad with mixed greens, almonds, and a vinaigrette dressing.

Snack 2: A serving of Savory Mushroom Jerky.

Dinner: Baked cod with a side of asparagus and wild rice.

Day 5:

Breakfast: Whole-grain toast with avocado and poached eggs.

Snack 1: A cup of green tea and Onion and Flaxseed Crackers.

Lunch: Chickpea and vegetable curry served with brown rice.

Snack 2: A small bowl of Mixed Berry Chia Delight.

Dinner: Grilled shrimp skewers with a mixed greens salad.

Day 6:

Breakfast: Chia seed pudding topped with sliced bananas and almonds.

Snack 1: Berry Spinach Smoothie.

Lunch: Turkey chili with beans and a side of whole-grain bread.

Snack 2: Spicy Roasted Chickpea Crunch.

Dinner: Lemon-garlic baked tilapia with steamed zucchini and couscous.

Day 7:

Breakfast: Blueberry and almond butter smoothie.

Snack 1: Pumpkin Seed and Goji Berry Trail Mix.

Lunch: Spinach and feta stuffed chicken breast with a quinoa and cucumber salad.

Snack 2: Vibrant Green Pea Hummus with whole-grain pita bread.

Dinner: Beef stir-fry with broccoli, bell peppers, and brown rice.

Day 8:

Breakfast: Buckwheat pancakes topped with a berry compote and a dollop of Greek yogurt.

Snack 1: A pear sliced and topped with a sprinkle of cinnamon.

Lunch: Arugula and roasted beet salad with goat cheese and walnuts, dressed with balsamic vinaigrette.

Snack 2: Carrot sticks and cucumber slices with Vibrant Green Pea Hummus.

Dinner: Lemon-herb roasted chicken thighs with a side of roasted Brussels sprouts and quinoa.

Day 9:

Breakfast: A smoothie bowl with spinach, frozen mango, coconut water, and topped with sliced kiwi and hemp seeds.

Snack 1: A small bowl of cottage cheese with pineapple chunks.

Lunch: Grilled vegetable and hummus sandwich on whole-grain bread.

Snack 2: A handful of raw almonds and dried cranberries.

Dinner: Garlic and olive oil spaghetti squash with a side of grilled asparagus.

Day 10:

Breakfast: Scrambled tofu with turmeric, black pepper, onions, and kale, served with whole-grain toast.

Snack 1: A banana with a tablespoon of almond butter.

Lunch: Quinoa and black bean stuffed bell peppers.

Snack 2: Crispy Kale and Nutritional Yeast Bites.

Dinner: Baked trout with a side salad of mixed greens, cherry tomatoes, and avocado.

Day 11:

Breakfast: Overnight oats with chia seeds, almond milk, and topped with fresh peach slices.

Snack 1: A small serving of Spicy Roasted Chickpea Crunch.

Lunch: A bowl of lentil soup with a side of mixed greens.

Snack 2: Sliced cucumber with a sprinkle of chili powder and lemon juice.

Dinner: Stir-fried tempeh with broccoli, bell peppers, and snow peas served over brown rice.

Day 12:

Breakfast: A frittata made with egg whites, spinach, mushrooms, and feta cheese.

Snack 1: An apple sliced and served with a small handful of pumpkin seeds.

Lunch: A tuna salad with mixed greens, cherry tomatoes, olives, and a hard-boiled egg.

Snack 2: Onion and Flaxseed Crackers with a slice of cheese.

Dinner: Moroccan spiced chickpea stew served with a side of couscous.

Day 13:

Breakfast: A parfait made with layers of Greek yogurt, granola, and mixed berries.

Snack 1: A small bowl of Mixed Berry Chia Delight.

Lunch: A turkey and avocado wrap with spinach and whole-grain tortilla.

Snack 2: A handful of Savory Mushroom Jerky.

Dinner: Grilled eggplant and zucchini stacks with tomato sauce and a sprinkle of Parmesan cheese.

Day 14:

Breakfast: A green smoothie with kale, pineapple, banana, and flaxseed.

Snack 1: A small serving of Pumpkin Seed and Goji Berry Trail Mix.

Lunch: A salad with mixed greens, grilled chicken, orange slices, and almonds with a citrus vinaigrette.

Snack 2: A few slices of pear with a schmear of ricotta cheese and a drizzle of honey.

Dinner: Pan-seared salmon with a side of sautéed green beans and a sweet potato.

Day 15:

Breakfast: Chia seed pudding made with coconut milk and topped with sliced kiwi and a sprinkle of flaxseeds.

Snack 1: A handful of blueberries and a few walnuts.

Lunch: Spinach and grilled chicken breast salad with avocado, pumpkin seeds, and a lemon-olive oil dressing.

Snack 2: Celery sticks with almond butter.

Dinner: Grilled tilapia with a mango salsa and a side of steamed green beans.

Day 16:

Breakfast: Whole-grain toast with smashed avocado and a side of cottage cheese.

Snack 1: A small bowl of Greek yogurt with a drizzle of honey and a sprinkle of cinnamon.

Lunch: Brown rice and black bean bowl with corn, tomatoes, and a dollop of guacamole.

Snack 2: A small apple with a slice of cheese.

Dinner: Turkey meatballs in a tomato sauce with zucchini noodles.

Day 17:

Breakfast: Omelet with tomatoes, onions, and spinach, served with a slice of whole-grain bread.

Snack 1: A pear and a small handful of almonds.

Lunch: Quinoa salad with roasted vegetables and feta cheese.

Snack 2: A few slices of cucumber and a hard-boiled egg.

Dinner: Baked cod with a side of roasted Brussels sprouts and sweet potatoes.

Day 18:

Breakfast: Protein smoothie with spinach, frozen berries, banana, and almond milk.

Snack 1: A small serving of hummus with carrot sticks.

Lunch: Whole-grain pita stuffed with mixed greens, grilled vegetables, and chickpeas.

Snack 2: A small bowl of cottage cheese with sliced tomatoes and a sprinkle of black pepper.

Dinner: Chicken stir-fry with a variety of vegetables served over brown rice.

Day 19:

Breakfast: Buckwheat porridge with sliced bananas and a drizzle of almond butter.

Snack 1: A small serving of trail mix with nuts and dried fruit.

Lunch: Lentil soup with a side of whole-grain bread and a mixed greens salad.

Snack 2: A few slices of bell pepper with guacamole.

Dinner: Grilled shrimp over a bed of mixed greens with a side of quinoa.

Day 20:

Breakfast: Toasted whole-grain English muffin with poached eggs and a side of sautéed spinach.

Snack 1: A small serving of roasted seaweed snacks.

Lunch: Tuna salad with mixed greens, cucumbers, and olives, dressed with olive oil and lemon.

Snack 2: A small serving of Spicy Roasted Chickpea Crunch.

Dinner: Vegetable curry with cauliflower, chickpeas, and peas served with a side of basmati rice.

Day 21:

Breakfast: Greek yogurt with a mix of sunflower seeds, chia seeds, and fresh raspberries.

Snack 1: A small serving of Mixed Berry Chia Delight.

Lunch: Turkey and spinach wrap with a side of mixed vegetable sticks.

Snack 2: A few slices of apple with a tablespoon of peanut butter.

Dinner: Baked lemon-pepper chicken breast with a side of asparagus and wild rice.

CHAPTER 9

LIFESTYLE FACTORS AND METABOLIC HEALTH

Lifestyle factors play a pivotal role in shaping our metabolic health, which in turn influences our overall well-being and disease risk, including cancer. Metabolic health refers to the optimal functioning of the body's chemical reactions and processes that maintain life. It encompasses the regulation of blood sugar, cholesterol levels, blood pressure, and the balance of hormones. When these processes are in harmony, the risk of metabolic diseases, including type 2 diabetes, heart disease, and certain types of cancer, is reduced. Lifestyle factors such as diet, physical activity, sleep, stress management, and social interactions are the keystones that can either support or undermine metabolic health.

Sleep, Stress, and Cancer Risk

Sleep and Metabolic Health

Sleep is a fundamental human need, as critical to health as diet and exercise. It is during sleep that the body undergoes repair and rejuvenation. Chronic sleep deprivation or poor-quality sleep can disrupt metabolic processes, leading to insulin resistance, increased appetite, and weight gain, all of which are risk factors for cancer. The relationship between sleep and cancer is complex and bidirectional. Not only can poor sleep contribute to the development of cancer, but the presence of cancer and its treatments can also impair sleep quality, creating a vicious cycle.

Adequate sleep supports the regulation of hormones such as leptin and ghrelin, which control appetite, and cortisol, which manages stress. Disruptions in these hormones can lead to metabolic imbalances, obesity, and an increased risk of cancer. For instance, breast cancer has been linked to low levels of melatonin, a hormone that regulates sleep-wake cycles and is produced during the dark. Exposure to light at night can suppress melatonin production, which is hypothesized to increase cancer risk.

Stress and Its Metabolic Implications

Stress is an inevitable aspect of life, but chronic stress can have profound effects on metabolic health. The body's stress response involves a cascade of hormones, including adrenaline and cortisol, which prepare the body for a 'fight or flight' reaction. While this response is beneficial in the short term, chronic activation can lead to a host of metabolic issues, such as high blood sugar and increased abdominal fat, which are linked to higher cancer risk.

The connection between stress and cancer is multifaceted. Stress can lead to unhealthy behaviors such as overeating, smoking, and sedentary habits, which further exacerbate metabolic dysfunction and cancer risk. Moreover, stress can directly affect cellular processes. For example, it can influence inflammation, DNA repair, and cell growth, all of which are critical in the development and progression of cancer.

The Importance of Community and Support

Social Connections and Metabolic Health

Humans are inherently social beings, and the quality of our social connections can significantly impact our health. A robust social network can provide emotional support, reduce stress, and encourage healthy behaviors, all of which contribute to better metabolic health and potentially lower cancer risk.

Community support can manifest in various ways, from family and friends to support groups and community organizations. These networks can offer practical help, such as assistance with healthcare appointments, as well as emotional support, which is crucial during challenging times. Social support can also foster a sense of belonging and purpose, which has been associated with better health outcomes, including improved survival rates for cancer patients.

Community, Behavior Change, and Cancer Prevention

Communities play a critical role in shaping health behaviors. They can create environments that promote physical activity, provide access to healthy foods, and support stress-reduction activities. For instance, community-led initiatives such as walking groups, community gardens, and meditation classes can encourage lifestyle changes that are conducive to metabolic health and cancer prevention.

Moreover, community support can enhance adherence to health-promoting behaviors. For example, a person is more likely to maintain an exercise routine if they are part of a group with similar goals. This social reinforcement can be particularly powerful for women, who often prioritize family and community well-being.

CHAPTER 10

BEYOND PREVENTION - A SUPPORTIVE JOURNEY

When Cancer Touches Your Life

Cancer is not a selective adversary; it can touch anyone's life, irrespective of their efforts in prevention. For women, this can be particularly challenging, given the unique interplay between hormones, reproductive health, and certain cancer risks. When cancer becomes a reality, the journey ahead requires not only courage but also a comprehensive understanding of how to navigate the complex world of cancer treatment. This chapter delves into the integration of metabolic approaches with traditional care and provides a guide for women to navigate treatments, ensuring that they are not passive recipients of health care but active, informed participants in their healing journey.

Integrating Metabolic Approaches with Traditional Care

The diagnosis of cancer often brings a sense of urgency and a rush towards conventional treatments such as surgery, chemotherapy, and radiation. These methods are the pillars of cancer treatment and have been the standard due to their effectiveness in reducing tumor burden. However, the integration of metabolic approaches into traditional care is emerging as a complementary strategy that may enhance treatment efficacy and improve quality of life.

Metabolic approaches to cancer care involve understanding and manipulating the metabolic dysfunctions that are characteristic of cancer cells. The Warburg effect, a phenomenon where cancer cells rely on glycolysis for energy production even in the presence of oxygen, is a prime example of such dysfunctions. By altering diet and exercise, the aim is to target these metabolic pathways that cancer cells depend on, potentially slowing disease progression and improving treatment outcomes.

Dietary Interventions

Diet plays a crucial role in metabolic therapy. A diet low in sugars and refined carbohydrates can reduce the availability of glucose to cancer cells, thus potentially inhibiting their growth. On the other hand, healthy fats and proteins can support the body's tissues and immune system. The ketogenic diet, which is high in fats and low in carbohydrates, is one such dietary approach that has gained attention for its potential to starve cancer cells while providing energy to normal cells through ketone bodies.

However, dietary interventions must be personalized. The nutritional needs of women with cancer can vary greatly depending on the type and stage of cancer, treatment modalities, and individual metabolic responses. Consulting with a dietitian who specializes in oncology can help tailor dietary approaches to each individual's needs, ensuring that the diet supports overall health and complements traditional treatments.

Exercise as a Complementary Therapy

Exercise is another pillar of metabolic therapy. Physical activity has been shown to improve insulin sensitivity, reduce inflammation, and enhance immune function—all of which are important in a body fighting cancer. Moreover, exercise can help combat fatigue, improve mood, and maintain muscle mass during cancer treatments, which can be physically and emotionally draining.

The type and intensity of exercise should be carefully considered and often need to be adjusted throughout the cancer journey. For instance, during active treatment, gentle forms of exercise like walking or yoga may be more appropriate, while more vigorous activity may be beneficial during recovery phases. Collaboration with a physical therapist or an exercise oncologist can help in designing an exercise program that is safe, effective, and adaptable to changing health statuses.

Navigating Treatments: A Woman's Guide

Navigating cancer treatments requires an understanding of the options available and how they may impact a woman's life. It's about making informed decisions that align with personal values, treatment goals, and quality of life considerations.

Understanding Treatment Options

Women should be encouraged to learn about the types of treatments offered for their specific type of cancer. This includes understanding how surgeries, chemotherapy, radiation, and newer treatments like immunotherapy or targeted therapies work, along with their potential side effects. Knowledge empowers women to ask informed questions and participate actively in treatment planning.

Side Effect Management

Managing side effects is a critical aspect of navigating cancer treatments. Women should be aware of the potential side effects of each treatment and have strategies in place to manage them. This includes both medical interventions and lifestyle modifications, such as dietary changes to manage nausea or exercise to reduce fatigue.

Emotional and Psychological Support

The emotional and psychological impact of cancer cannot be overstated. Women may experience a range of emotions from fear and anxiety to depression and anger. Seeking support from mental health professionals, support groups, or community resources can be invaluable. Mind-body practices such as meditation, mindfulness, and counseling can also play a significant role in managing the psychological challenges of cancer.

Advocacy and Communication

Effective communication with healthcare providers is essential. Women should feel empowered to advocate for themselves, ask questions, and express their concerns and preferences. Bringing a family member or friend to appointments can help in understanding and remembering the information provided by the healthcare team.

Long-Term Planning

Cancer treatment is not just about the immediate fight; it's also about long-term health planning. This includes discussions about fertility preservation before treatment, the management of menopausal symptoms, and the monitoring for long-term side effects or secondary cancers.

Survivorship and Thriving

Survivorship, in the context of cancer, begins at diagnosis and continues through treatment and beyond. It encompasses the physical, psychosocial, and economic issues of cancer, from diagnosis until the end of life. Thriving, however, goes a step further—it's not just about survival but about flourishing despite the challenges that come with a cancer journey. This chapter is dedicated to understanding how women can not only survive cancer but also thrive after their treatment, with a particular focus on the role of nutrition and exercise in recovery.

The Role of Nutrition in Recovery

Nutrition plays a pivotal role in the recovery phase of a cancer survivor. After the arduous journey of treatments such as chemotherapy, radiation, or surgery, the body is often depleted and in need of vital nutrients to rebuild tissue, regain strength, and boost the immune system. A well-considered diet can help mitigate the side effects of treatment, enhance the body's ability to repair itself, and improve overall well-being.

During recovery, the metabolic demands of the body are often higher. The right mix of macronutrients—proteins, carbohydrates, and fats—is crucial. Proteins are particularly important as they are the building blocks for repair. Women should aim for high-quality protein sources, such as lean meats, fish, eggs, and legumes, to aid in the repair of tissues damaged by cancer treatment.

Carbohydrates are the body's primary energy source, and choosing the right kind is essential. Complex carbohydrates, found in whole grains, fruits, and vegetables, provide a steady release of energy, as well as vital fiber, which can help manage issues such as constipation often caused by pain medications.

Fats should not be overlooked, especially those rich in omega-3 fatty acids, which have been shown to have anti-inflammatory properties. Sources like salmon, flaxseeds, and walnuts can be beneficial.

Micronutrients—vitamins and minerals—also play a significant role. For example, antioxidants help combat oxidative stress, which can be heightened after cancer treatments. However, it's important to note that high doses of antioxidants should be avoided during treatment, as they can interfere with the effectiveness of chemotherapy and radiation.

Hydration is another key aspect of nutrition in recovery. Adequate fluid intake is essential for all bodily functions, including nutrient transport and waste removal.

Exercise in Recovery

Exercise is another cornerstone of thriving in survivorship. It can help rebuild strength and stamina, reduce the risk of cancer recurrence, and improve quality of life. However, the approach to exercise post-cancer treatment should be gentle and progressive.

Starting with low-intensity activities, such as walking or gentle yoga, can help survivors regain mobility and flexibility. Gradually, as strength and endurance improve, the intensity of exercises can be increased. Strength training is particularly important as it helps rebuild muscle mass and bone density, which can be adversely affected by cancer treatments.

Cardiovascular exercise also has its place in recovery. It can improve heart health, reduce fatigue, and enhance mood. Activities like cycling, swimming, or even dancing can be enjoyable ways for survivors to incorporate aerobic exercise into their routine.

It's important for survivors to work with healthcare providers to create an exercise plan tailored to their individual needs and limitations. The goal is to find a sustainable and enjoyable form of exercise that supports recovery and overall health.

Stories of Hope: Women's Experiences with a Metabolic Approach

The true testament to the power of a metabolic approach to cancer comes from the stories of women who have lived it. These narratives not only provide inspiration but also invaluable insights into the practical application of nutrition and exercise in the journey to recovery.

One such story is of a woman who, after battling breast cancer, adopted a ketogenic diet under the guidance of her nutritionist. She reported not only a significant improvement in her energy levels but also a newfound sense of control over her health.

Another survivor found solace and strength in exercise. After her treatment for ovarian cancer, she began a gentle yoga practice. Over time, she credits this practice with helping her regain not just physical strength but also mental clarity and emotional stability.

These stories underscore the importance of individualized approaches. What works for one person may not work for another, and the metabolic approach to cancer is not a one-size-fits-all solution. It's about finding the right balance of nutrition and exercise that works for each woman's unique body and circumstances.

CONCLUSION

The journey through cancer is profound and transformative. It is a path marked by challenges and revelations, despair and hope. For women, this journey is navigated with the added complexity of gender-specific health concerns and societal roles that often place them as primary caregivers, even as they need care themselves. The metabolic approach to cancer for women is not just about managing a disease; it's about embracing a lifestyle that fosters resilience, promotes healing, and empowers women to take charge of their health.

In the preceding chapters, we have explored the intricate relationship between metabolism and cancer, the critical role of nutrition and exercise in prevention and recovery, and the inspiring stories of women who have turned their cancer battles into journeys of profound self-discovery and healing. As we draw this book to a close, it's essential to crystallize the key takeaways and reflect on the broader implications of adopting a metabolic approach to cancer.

The Metabolic Paradigm

At its core, the metabolic approach to cancer challenges traditional views by positing that cancer is not just a genetic disease but a metabolic one, influenced by the body's energy production and nutrient utilization. This paradigm shift opens up new avenues for prevention and treatment, emphasizing the importance of diet and lifestyle choices in modulating cancer risk and progression. For women, this means that the power to influence their health outcomes lies not only in the hands of their healthcare providers but also in their own hands, through the daily choices they make about what to eat and how to move.

Nutrition as a Pillar of Health

Nutrition has emerged as a pillar of health in the fight against cancer. A diet that is rich in whole foods, low in processed sugars, and balanced in macronutrients can support the body's natural defenses and create an environment less conducive to cancer growth. For women recovering from cancer, nutrition becomes even more critical as the body needs a plethora of nutrients to repair and rebuild. The science of nutrition is complex, but the message is simple: what women eat can be a powerful ally in their cancer journey.

Exercise as a Catalyst for Recovery

Exercise is the catalyst that can accelerate recovery and enhance quality of life. It's not just about burning calories; it's about building a body that is strong, resilient, and capable of withstanding the rigors of cancer treatment and the stresses of everyday life. Exercise can help mitigate some of the most challenging side effects of cancer treatments, such as fatigue, muscle atrophy, and depression. For women, incorporating exercise into their recovery plan can also provide a sense of normalcy and control at a time when life seems anything but normal.

The Power of Personal Stories

Throughout this book, we have woven in the personal stories of women who have faced cancer head-on and have found hope and healing through a metabolic approach. These narratives are more than just anecdotes; they are the lived experiences that validate the science and provide a roadmap for others. They remind us that behind every statistic and every study are real women with real stories of courage and triumph.

Challenges and Considerations

While the metabolic approach offers hope, it's important to acknowledge the challenges and considerations that come with it. Access to healthy foods and safe spaces for exercise, the ability to take time for self-care, and the financial resources to support a health-focused lifestyle are not equally available to all women. There is also the risk of information overload and the confusion that can come from the myriad of dietary and exercise regimens touted as cancer-preventive or curative. Navigating these challenges requires support, education, and sometimes, guidance from professionals.

Looking Ahead

As we look to the future, the metabolic approach to cancer holds promise not just for individual women but for the healthcare system and society at large. It represents a shift towards a more holistic, preventative model of health care that empowers patients and prioritizes wellness over disease. It's a call to action for researchers, healthcare providers, and policymakers to invest in further research, education, and infrastructure that support the metabolic approach to health.

Empowerment Through Education

Education is empowerment. By understanding the metabolic underpinnings of cancer, women can make informed decisions about their health. This book aims to be a resource that educates, enlightens, and empowers women to take an active role in their health journey. It's a testament to the strength and resilience of women who have battled cancer and a guide for those who seek to prevent or are currently fighting the disease.

Final Thoughts

In conclusion, the metabolic approach to cancer for women is more than a dietary or exercise plan; it's a philosophy of living. It's about making choices that nourish the body, engage the mind, and uplift the spirit. It's about not just surviving but thriving, with vitality and joy. The path to wellness is as individual as the women who walk it, but the destination is the same—a life lived with health, grace, and empowerment.

As readers turn the final page of this book, it is hoped that they feel equipped with knowledge, inspired by stories, and motivated to embark on their own journeys of health and healing. The metabolic approach to cancer is a path paved with challenges, but it is also lined with hope. It's a journey that many women have taken and one that many more will take. Together, through the collective wisdom shared in these pages, women can support each other in not just surviving cancer but in thriving in the face of it.

Printed in the USA
CPSIA information can be obtained
at www.ICGtesting.com
LVHW012359010424
776064LV00024B/483

9 798866 963874